CONTENTS

THE PROPER FASTING

Take advice the right way

Solid evidences from the Islamic Approach

Book 1

Djemoi BENDAHMANE

"Fasting is a shield*..."

The prophet Muhammad

to my beloved wife

to my childrens Iyad & AbdalKafi

INTRODUCTION

Today, fasting in its various forms has become an important component in the lives of individuals, who seek to preserve their health from all diseases and ills. This is confirmed by studies day after day, where fasting represents an immune system against what may affect the human body.

Through my experience with fasting for years and through my research in this field, it became clear to me that there is a great scientific interest in fasting according to its Islamic form. Most studies found that there is a strong correlation between this form of fasting and the prevention of diseases.

The true framework for the proper Islamic fasting is structured within two main sources: the Quran and all the sayings and actions of the Messenger of Allah "Muhammad".

Within the following pages, I will present a very simplified content and structure of this fast with attention to most of its components on the one hand. On the other hand, I will try to highlight the forms and the main motives behind the adoption of 1.8 billion people to this approach, in a way that allows the reader to understand and understand the content.

The pages of the book aim to guide you, looking step by step to judge and with conviction on all the beliefs and ideas marketed about fasting in our world, and that fasting according to the Allah's method is simple and it is the right choice for the prevention of diseases, weight loss, psychological comfort and sexual force ... etc.

CHAPTER I

The fasting is a pillar

F asting is another unique moral and spiritual characteristic of Islam. The Arabic word 'sawm' is used for fasting. The term 'to fast' literary means 'to refrain' (absolute abstention and self-restraint). Fasting for Muslims is sacred because it imposed upon them by order of Allah through the Quran (Allah's Book) since more than fourteen centuries.

According to Islamic legislation fasting means abstention from drinking, eating and restraint of sexual intercourse, as a form of worship to Allah, being from dawn to sunset.

The Quran and the Prophet Muhammad gives us a great framework of fasting, and show us the main meaning, the kinds, the proper way and the greater purpose of fasting.

Allah says in the Quran:

> *"O you who believe! Observing As-Saum (the fasting) is prescribed for you as it was prescribed for those before you, that you may become Al-Muttaqun (the pious)."* (Quran 2:183)

> *"[Observing Saum (fasts)] for a fixed number of days, but if any of you is ill or on a journey, the same number (should be made up) from other days. And as for those who can fast with difficulty, (e.g. an old man, etc.), they have (a choice either to fast or) to feed a Miskin (poor person) (for every day). But whoever does good of his own accord, it is better for him. And that you fast, it is better for you if only you know."* (Quran 2:184)

> *"The month of Ramadan in which was revealed the Quran, a guidance for mankind*

and clear proofs for the guidance and the criterion (between right and wrong). So whoever of you sights (the crescent on the first night of) the month (of Ramadan i.e. is present at his home), he must observe Saum (fasts) that month, and whoever is ill or on a journey, the same number [of days which one did not observe Saum (fasts) must be made up] from other days. Allah intends for you ease, and He does not want to make things difficult for you. (He wants that you) must complete the same number (of days), and that you must magnify Allah [i.e. to say Takbir (Allahu-Akbar; Allah is the Most Great) on seeing the crescent of the months of Ramadan and Shawwal] for having guided you so that you may be grateful to Him." (Quran 2:185)

"It is made lawful for you to have sexual relations with your wives on the night of As-Saum (the fasts). They are Libas [i.e. body cover, or screen, or Sakan, (i.e. you enjoy the pleasure of living with her), for you and you are the same for them. Allah knows that you used to deceive yourselves, so He turned to you (accepted your repentance) and forgave you. So now have sexual relations with them and seek that which Allah

has ordained for you (offspring), and eat and drink until the white thread (light) of dawn appears to you distinct from the black thread (darkness of night), then complete your Saum (fast) till the nightfall. And do not have sexual relations with them (your wives) while you are in I'tikaf (i.e. confining oneself in a mosque for prayers and invocations leaving the worldly activities) in the mosques. These are the limits (set) by Allah, so approach them not. Thus does Allah make clear His Ayat (proofs, evidences, lessons, signs, revelations, verses, laws, legal and illegal things, Allah's set limits, orders, etc.) to mankind that they may become Al-Muttaqun (the pious)." (Quran 2:187)

And according to the Messenger of Allah (Muhammad) said:

"Islam is built on five (pillars): bearing witness that there is no god except Allaah and that Muhammad is the Messenger of Allaah, establishing prayer, paying zakaah, Hajj and fasting Ramadaan." Al-Bukhaari (8) and Muslim (16).

Islam is an act of duties and is subordination to the command of God. This means that whoever came to these five pillars has completed his Islam. Islam, like the house, can only be made by its pillars.

This Hadith from the Prophet Muhammad indicates that Ramadan must be fast, and that it is one of the pillars and foundations upon which the Islam of the individual is based. God commanded His slaves in His wisdom for great reasons.

You can imagine that a Muslim loses the status of Islam if he abandons the fast of Ramadan under any excuse not mentioned by Islamic legislation.

CHAPTER II

Fasting types

S ome believe Ramadan fasting is the only fast one in Islam, but the truth is otherwise. According to the Islamic legislation, there are four type of fasting: Obligatory fasting, Fasting as expiation (Kaffarah), Fasting to fulfill a vow (Nadhr) and voluntary fasting.

1. Obligatory fasting

Ramadan fasting (the ninth month of the Muslim

lunar calendar) is an obligation for all Muslims, which all are required to abstain during daylight hours from eating, drinking, or engaging in sexual activity.

With increasing awareness of their spiritual and physical needs, Muslims have become more aware of Allah's presence and are grateful for the existence of Allah's judgments in their lives.

Fasting in Ramadan is required of all Muslims, except sick, children or elderly, who travel, women who are menstruating, or have just given birth... In such cases and others, one can spend the days of fasting later.

2. Fasting as expiation (Kaffarah)

The word 'expiation" means: reparation; expiation from wrongdoing; atonement; penance.

Allah has set limits prescribed in his Quran or mentioned by the Prophet Muhammad, Allah says in the Quran:

"These are the limits of Allah, which He

makes plain for the people who have knowledge." (Quran 2:230)

If a Muslim transgresses Allah's limits, it should to free himself from its, he should be subject to certain penalties prescribed by Allah and the messenger such as Expiation, Ransom, blood-money and others. One of the most significant ways of how a person can free himself is to observe fast, the following is an explication of that:

2.1 Fast is random to removing hair in Hajj or 'Umrah

Upon making Ihraam for Hajj or 'Umrah, there are certain things that are forbidden as long as one is in the state of Ihraam (Hajj or 'Umrah). One of these thing is removing hair of head. If a Muslim does that, he must free himself from this transgressing, as Allah says in Quran:

"And perform properly (i.e. all the ceremonies according to the ways of Prophet Muhammad), the Hajj and 'Umrah (i.e. the pilgrimage to Makkah) for Allah. But if you are pre-

vented (from completing them), sacrifice a Hady (animal, i.e. a sheep, a cow, or a camel, etc.) such as you can afford, and do not shave your heads until the Hady reaches the place of sacrifice. And whosoever of you is ill or has an ailment in his scalp (necessitating shaving), he must pay a Fidyah (ransom) of either observing Saum (fasts) (three days) or giving Sadaqah (charity - feeding six poor persons) or offering sacrifice (one sheep) ..." (Quran 2:196)

2.2 If the pilgrim cannot find or afford a Hady (sacrificial animal) in Hajj

If the pilgrim is performing a Hajj, it is required to him to offer a Hady, which is to be slaughtered on the day of An-Nahr (slaughter) (the 10th of Thul-Hijjah) and distribute it among the poor of Makkah. If he cannot find or afford this Hady, it is must to him to fasts, as Allah says in Quran:

"...Then if you are in safety and whosoever performs the 'Umrah in the months of Hajj, before (performing) the Hajj, he must slaughter a Hady such as he can afford, but if he cannot afford it, he should observe

Saum (fasts) three days during the Hajj and seven days after his return (to his home), making ten days in all. This is for him whose family is not present at Al-Masjid-al-Haram (i.e. non-resident of Makkah). And fear Allah much and know that Allah is Severe in punishment. " (Quran 2:196)

2.3 If a Muslim killed a Muslim by mistake

In this case, the expiation for killing a Muslim by accident is to free a slave and a compensation (blood money, i.e. Diya) must be given to the deceased's family, If that is not possible then it is must to fasting for two consecutive months.

Allah says in Quran:

"It is not for a believer to kill a believer except (that it be) by mistake, and whosoever kills a believer by mistake, (it is ordained that) he must set free a believing slave and a compensation (blood money, i.e. Diya) be given to the deceased's family, unless they remit it. If the deceased belonged to a people at war with you and he was a believer; the freeing of a believing slave (is prescribed), and if

he belonged to a people with whom you have a treaty of mutual alliance, compensation (blood money - Diya) must be paid to his family, and a believing slave must be freed. And whoso finds this (the penance of freeing a slave) beyond his means, he must fast for two consecutive months in order to seek repentance from Allah. And Allah is Ever All-Knowing, All-Wise." (Quran 4:92)

2.4 The expiation for breaking an oath

The Muslim should protect his oath and not swear oaths willy-nilly concerning matters that do not deserve to have the oath sworn. In this matter, Allah described the Fasting as one of the way for expiating the oath.

And this as stated in the following verse, Allah says:

"Allah will not punish you for what is unintentional in your oaths, but He will punish you for your deliberate oaths; for its expiation (a deliberate oath) feed ten Masakin (poor persons), on a scale of the average of that with which you feed your own families;

13

or clothe them; or manumit a slave. But whosoever cannot afford (that), then he should fast for three days. That is the expiation for the oaths when you have sworn. And protect your oaths (i.e. do not swear much). Thus Allah make clear to you His Ayat (proofs, evidences, verses, lessons, signs, revelations, etc.) that you may be grateful." (Quran 5:89)

2.5 The expiation for killing games in a state of Ihram for Hajj or 'Umrah (pilgrimage)

Similarly, killing games during the Hajj or 'Umrah needs expiation. Fasting is prescribed as one of the way for expiation.

Allah says in Quran:

" O you who believe! Kill not game while you are in a state of Ihram for Hajj or 'Umrah (pilgrimage), and whosoever of you kills it intentionally, the penalty is an offering, brought to the Ka'bah, of an eatable animal (i.e. sheep, goat, cow, etc.) equivalent to the one he killed, as adjudged by two just men among you; or, for expiation, he should feed Masakin (poor persons), or its equivalent in Saum (fasting), that he may taste the

heaviness (punishment) of his deed. Allah has forgiven what is past, but whosoever commits it again, Allah will take retribution from him. And Allah is All-Mighty, All-Able of Retribution." (Quran 5:95)

2.6 The expiation for Az-zihar

Az-Zihar is the saying of a husband of his wife 'you are to me like the back of my mother (i.e. unlawful for me). Fasting has been prescribed as one of the ways for expiation.

Allah in the Quran said:

"Those among you who make their wives unlawful (Az-Zihar) to them by saying to them "You are like my mother's back." They cannot be their mothers. None can be their mothers except those who gave them birth. And verily, they utter an ill word and a lie. And verily, Allah is Oft-Pardoning, Oft-Forgiving. " (Quran 58:2)

"And those who make unlawful to them (their wives) (by Az-Zihar) and wish to free themselves from what they uttered, (the penalty) in that case (is) the freeing of a slave

before they touch each other. That is an admonition to you (so that you may not return to such an ill thing). And Allah is All-Aware of what you do. " (Quran 58:3)

"And he who finds not (the money for freeing a slave) must fast two successive months before they both touch each other. And for him who is unable to do so, he should feed sixty of Miskin (poor). That is in order that you may have perfect Faith in Allah and His Messenger. These are the limits set by Allah. And for disbelievers, there is a painful torment. " (Quran 58:4)

2.7 The (Kafara) expiation for one who has sex with his wife during the day of Ramadan

A Muslim who has sex with his wife during the day of Ramadan, his fast becomes null and void. On the other hand, he is required to expiate his sin either by freeing a slave, failing that he should observe fast for two consecutive months, failing that he must feed sixty poor people. Moreover, he has to follow the mentioned order of expiation in case of failing short of doing any of the three ways.

This is the opinion of the majority of Muslim scholars. This opinion is based on a narration reported by Al-Bukhari and Muslim from Abu Hurayrah:

> *"A person came to The Messenger of Allah (Muhammad) and said: 'O Messenger of Allah! I am doomed'. The Prophet, said: 'What has brought about your ruin?' The person said: 'I had a sexual enter course with my wife during the month of Ramadan (i.e. during the day)'. Upon this the Prophet said: "Can you find a slave to set him free? He said: 'No'. The Prophet said: "Can you observe fast for two consecutive months? He said: 'No'. The Prophet said: "Can you provide food for sixty poor people?" He said: 'No'. Abu Hurayrah said: 'While we were sitting with the Prophet a large basket full of dates was produced to the Prophet . So, the Prophet said: "Where is the inquirer?" He said: 'Me'. The Prophet said: "Take this and give it as charity."* Al-Bukhaari (1936) and Muslim (81)

3. Fasting to fulfill a vow (Nadhr)

In Arabic, you say: I vowed so: if you enjoined an order on yourself.

In Islam, the vow is: to commit yourself to something for Allah.

The Muslim be careful with regard to the issue of vows, because making a vow to Allah to do something or to refrain from something is not a light matter. The one who makes a vow is enjoined to fulfil it and is subject to a threat of punishment if he breaks that vow.

The Messenger of Allah (Muhammad) said:

> *"Whoever vows to obey Allah, let him obey Him. Whoever vows to disobey Allah, let him not disobey Him."* Muslim (106).

4. Voluntary fasting

Firstly, Allah made voluntary fasting a good thing for those who did it. Where he said in Quran:

> *"... And whoever volunteers excess - it is better for him. But to fast is best for you, if you only knew."* (Quran 2:184)

Secondly, the Messenger of Islam (Muhammad) encourages and motivates the Muslims to do this fast:

> *Abu Umaamah, said that he went to the Messenger of Allah and said to him, "Order me to do something that I take from you." The Prophet said: "Observe fasting, for there is nothing like it (i.e. in reward)."*

In another narration,

> *Abu Umaamah said that he went to the Messenger of Allah and said to him, "Order me to do something that I may take from you." The Prophet said: "Observe fasting, for it has no equivalent."*

This is really great and very important.

Well, according to Islamic legislation, voluntary fasting is two kinds:

4.1 Absolute voluntary fasting

Not restricted to any particular time or circumstances. The Muslim may observe a voluntary fast on any day of the year that he wishes, except those which are known to be forbidden.

The Prophet Muhammad strongly calls for absolute voluntary fasting; there are many narrations that confirm this, such as:

> *Abu Umaamah said that he went to the Messenger of Allah and said to him, "Order me to do something that I may take from you." The Prophet said: "Observe fasting, for it has no equivalent."*

4.2 Designated voluntary fasting

Is restricted to a certain times or circumstances according to sources. Designated voluntary fasting is better than the absolute voluntary fasting; there are many kinds of this fasting, as the following:

a. Fasting for six days in Shawwal, the month after Ramadan

Abu Ayyoob reported that the Prophet Muhammad said:

> *"Whoever fasts Ramadan and follows it with six days of Shawwaal, it will be as if he fasted for a lifetime."*

b. Fasting the first nine days in Dhul-Hijjah

Dhul-Hijjah is the (the Month of Hajj) is the 12th month of the Islamic lunar Calendar.

One of the wives of the Prophet Muhammad said:

> *"Allah's Messenger used to fast the [first] nine days of Dhul-Hijjah, the day of `Ashurah, and three days of each month."*

> *c. Fasting the Day of Arafah (9th day of Dhul-Hijjah of the lunar Islamic Calendar) for those who are not performing Hajj*

It was narrated from Abu Qatadah that the Messenger of Allah was asked about fasting on the day of 'Arafah and he said:

> *"It expiates for the past and coming years."*
> Muslim (1162)

According to another report:

> *"I ask Allah that it may expiate for (the sins of) the year that comes before it and the year that comes after it."*

d. Fasting the month of Muharram (the 1st Islamic calendar month)

Abu Huraira reported: The Messenger of Allah, said:

> *"The best fasting after Ramadan is the month of Allah Muharram, and the best prayer after the obligatory prayer is prayer at night."* Muslim (1163)

e. The fast of Ashurah (Fasting on the ninth and tenth days or tenth and eleventh days of the month of Muharram)

Fasting the day of Ashurah does expiate for the past year, because the Prophet said:

"...Thereafter the Prophet said: Fasting three days every month and that of Ramadan every year is a perpetual fasting. I seek from Allah that fasting on the day of 'Arafah may atone for the sins of the preceding and the coming years, and I seek from Allah that fasting on the day of Ashurah may atone for the sins of the preceding year." Muslim (1162)

And, Ibn Abbas reported that when Allah's Messenger came to Medina, he found the Jews observing the fast on the day of Ashurah. They (the Jews) were asked about it and they said:

"It is the day on which Allah granted victory to Moses and (his people) Bani Isra'il

over the Pharaoh and we observe fast out of gratitude to Him. Upon this the Messenger of Allah said: We have a closer connection with Moses than you have", and he commanded to observe fast on this day.

f. Fast on the month of Sha'ban

Sha'ban is the eighth month of the Islamic calendar. The month before Ramadan.

One of the great things in Islam is fasting the month of Sha'ban given the great benefits in it. Many of the narrations about the Prophet Muhammad showed the importance of fasting in this month:

A'isha, the Mother of the Believers, reported:

"that the Messenger of Allah used to fast (so continuously) that we said that he would not break, and did not fast at all till we said that he would not fast. And I did not see the Messenger of Allah completing the fast of a month, but that of Ramadan, and I did not see him fasting more in any other month

than that of Sha'ban". Muslim (1156)

Also, Usamah bin Zaid said:

> *"I said: 'O Messenger of Allah, I do not see you fasting any month as much as Shaban.' He said: 'That is a month to which people do not pay much attention, between Rajab and Ramadan. It is a month in which the deeds are taken up to the Lord of the worlds, and I like that my deeds be taken up when I am fasting."* An-Nasaa'i (2357)

g. Fasting on Mondays and Thursdays

One of the best fast is on Monday and Thursday every week. This is recommended by the prophet Muhammad.

Abu Qatadah reported: The Messenger of Allah was asked about fasting on Mondays. He said

"That is the day on which I was born and the day on which I received Revelation." Muslim (1162)

And, Usamah bin Zaid said:

"I said: 'O Messenger of Allah, sometimes you fast, and you hardly ever break your hardly ever fast, except two days which, if you are fasting, you include them in your fast, and if you are not fasting, then you fast them on your own.' He said: 'Which two days?' I said: 'Monday and Thursday.' He said: 'Those are two days in which deeds are shown to the Lord of the worlds, and I like my deeds to be shown (to Him) when I am fasting." Sunan an-Nasa'I (2358)

h. Fast three days of every month

We can distinguish two parts of this type of fasting as follow:

1 # fasting three days of every month without specifying

It was narrated that Abu Hurayrah said:

"My close friend (the Prophet) advised me to do three things which I will not give up until I die: fasting three days of each month, praying Duhaa and going to sleep after Witr". Al-Bukhaari (1124) and Muslim (721)

And,

Abu Murra, the freed slave of Umm Hani, narrated on the authority of Abu Darda':

"My Friend (the Prophet) instructed me in three (acts), and I would never abandon them as long as I live. (And these three things are): Three fasts during every month, the forenoon prayer, and this that I should not sleep till I have observed the Witr prayer". Muslim (722)

2 # fasting on the three white days of every lunar month

The white days are the thirteenth, fourteenth and fifteenth of every lunar month, they were named with this name because the moon becomes full on them and the light becomes strong which makes their nights are completely luminous.

Abu Dharr said:

> *The Messenger of Allah said to me: "If you fast any part of the month, then fast the thirteenth, fourteenth and fifteenth."* Al-Tirmidhi (761)

i. Fasting one day and skipping the other day in days other than Ramadan (Fasting of Prophet David)

Whoever has a great desire to fast, has strength, wanted to increase fasting to previous types, he fasts one day, and breaks one day, and he does not fast more than that, because this is the highest degree of volunteer fasting for those who have the power and ability to do so.

In the narration of Abdullah ibn 'Amr that the Prophet Muhammad said:

> *"The best fasting is the fast of Dawood (The Prophet David): he used to fast one day and not the next."*

j. Fasting for those who cannot afford marriage

Urge Islam to marry because it preserves man's nature and existence. But whoever cannot afford the marriage and its costs, it gives him a great solution is fasting.

Abdullah b. Mas'ud reported that Allah's Messenger said to us:

> *"O young men, those among you who can support a wife should marry, for it restrains eyes (from casting evil glances) and preserves one from immorality; but he who cannot afford it should observe fast for it is a means of controlling the sexual desire."* Muslim (1400)

DJEMOI BENDAHMANE

CHAPTER III

The days when fasting is not permissible (Forbidden)

1. Fasting the days of Eid al-Fitr and Eid al Adha

In Islam there are two Eids (festivals), Eid al Fitr "festival of breaking the fast", also referred to as the smaller Eid, and Eid al Adha "Festival of the Sacrifice" which is the bigger Eid. Eid al Fitr celebrates the end of the holy month of Ramadan (month of obligatory fasting), and this Eid is announced at the beginning of the 10th month of the Islamic calendar called Shawwal, which follows the month of Ramadan. The sighting of the moon is therefore important in announcing the start of a new lunar month.

Muslims celebrate Eid al Fitr to show thankfulness to Allah for allowing them to finish and be able to fulfill their obligation by fasting, completing good deeds in the sacred month.

Eid al Adha "Festival of the Sacrifice" is celebrated on the end of the Hajj (annual pilgrimage to Makkah) on the 10th day of Dhul-Hijjah (the last month of the Islamic calendar). During this celebration, Muslims commemorate and remember Abraham's trials, by themselves slaughtering an animal such as a sheep, camel, or goat.

The meat from the sacrifice is mostly given away to others people. One-third is eaten by immediate family, one-third is given away to friends, and one-third is donated to the poor of believers.

It is forbidden to fast on the first day of Eid al Fitr, and on all four days of Eid al Adha. This is because those days are the days to eat, drink, share and celebrate the blessings that God has granted us.

There are several narrations related to this prohibition:

> *"A'isha (the Prophet Muhammad's wife) said that the Prophet forbade to observe fast on two days-the day of Fitr and the day of Adha."* Muslim (1140)

And, Abu Ubaid, the freed slave of Ibn Azhar, reported:

I observed El Eid along with Umar b. Al-Khattab. He came (out in an open space) and prayed and (after) completing it addressed the people and said:

> *"The Messenger of Allah has forbidden the observing of fast on these two days. One is the day of Fitr (at the end of your fasts), and the second one, the day when you eat (the meat) of your sacrifices."* Muslim (1137)

Also, Nubaisha al-Hudhali reported Allah's Messenger as saying:

"The days of Tashriq are the days of eating and drinking." Muslim (1141)

The days of tashriq are the 11th, 12th, 13th of the month Dhul-Hijjah, which are the 2nd, 3rd and 4th days of Eid al-Adha.

The wisdom of not offering fast on the day of Eid is that the day of Eid Al-Fitr is the day of breaking the fast from Ramadan, and Ramadan cannot be specified [singled out] except by breaking the fast [not fasting] on the day of Eid.

With regard to Eid Al-Adha, it is because it is the day of sacrifice, and if people were to fast on this day, they would have acted differently from what Allah loves and ordered us to do in His saying:

"So eat of them and feed the miserable and poor." (Quran 22:28)

2. Fasting one or two days before Ramadan

Abu Huraira reported Allah's Messenger as saying:

"Do not anticipate Ramadan by fasting one or two days before it begins, but if a man habitually fasts, then let him fast." Muslim (1082)

With this narration and others from the Prophet Muhammad, clearly indicate that it is not permissible to anticipate Ramadan by fasting one or two days before it begins.

CHAPTER IV

The days when fasting is prohibited (disliked)

1. Fasting for a lifetime

The prophet Muhammad prohibited of Fasting for a lifetime, and the better is fast one day and break on the other day.

'Abdullah b. 'Amr b. al-'As reported that the Messenger of Allah was informed that he could stand up for (prayer) throughout the night and observe fast every day so long as he lived. Thereupon the

Messenger of Allah said:

"Is it you who said this? I said to him: Messenger of Allah, it is I who said that. Thereupon the Messenger of Allah said: You are not capable enough to do so. Observe fast and break it; sleep and stand for prayer, and observe fast for three days during the month; for every good is multiplied ten times and this is like fasting for ever. I said: Messenger of Allah. I am capable of doing more than this. Thereupon he said: Fast one day and do not fast for the next two days. I said: Messenger of Allah, I have the strength to do more than that. The Prophet, said: Fast one day and break on the other day. That is known as the fasting of David and that is the best fasting. I said: I am capable of doing more than this. Thereupon the Messenger of Allah said: There is nothing better than this. 'Abdullah b. 'Amr said: Had I accepted the three days (fasting during every month) as the Messenger of Allah had said, it would have been dearer to me than my family and my property."
Muslim (1159)

2. Fasting on the day of Arafah for the pilgrim in Hajj

The day of Arafah is the ninth day of Dhu'l-Hijjah (the last day of Hajj). Fasting on this day is a recommended fast for those who are not performing Hajj. (see Ch.3).

During his Hajj, the Prophet Muhammad did not fast.

> *"Umm al-Fadl bint- al-Harith reported that some people argued about the fasting of the Messenger of Allah on the day of 'Arafah. Some of them said that he had been fasting, whereas the others said that he had not been fasting. I sent a cup of milk to him while he was riding his camel at 'Arafah and he drank it."* Muslim (1123)

3. Single out Friday or Saturday for fasting

Singling out a day for observing a voluntary fasting is permissible, except to single out Friday or Saturday. It is hates fasting on Friday or Saturday alone, this is what the Prophet has recommended.

Abu Huraira reported the Messenger of Allah as

saying:

"I heard the Prophet say: "No one of you should fast on Friday, unless he fasts (a day) before it or after it." Muslim (1144)

And, narrated As-Samma' sister of Abdullah ibn Busr:

The Prophet said: "Do not fast on Saturday except what has been made obligatory on you; and if one of you can get nothing but a grape skin or a piece of wood from a tree, he should chew it." Sunan Abi Dawud (2421)

It is disliked to single out Saturday for fasting, because the Jews venerate Saturday.

CHAPTER V

Why do Muslims Fast?

I n the actual world, people do fast for many reasons, based upon on their religious, intellectual, cultural, financial, medical, political and social beliefs. Some of these reasons are:

- Promotes Blood Sugar

- Promotes Better Health by Fighting Inflammatio

- Enhance Heart Health by Improving Blood Pressure, Triglycerides and Cholesterol Levels

- Boost Brain Functio

 - Weight Loss

- Muscle Strength

- Cancers Prevention

- Training of the mind and the body to endure and harden up against all hardships...etc.

In addition to these and other reasons, the Muslims fast with a desire to reach near to Allah and to earn Allah's blessings and rewards. Muslims' reasons to do fast are very many and have been explained in the Quran and in the sayings and deeds of the Prophet Muhammad.

The benefits and virtues of fasting in Islam motivate everyone to observe fasting. These can achieved thought the true fasting (the fast based on the Islamic legislation).

Some of these reasons are:

1. Fasting is a way to achieve and develop Taqwa

Taqwa is the ultimate virtue of fasting, it is means fear of Allah and done all duties he ordered. Allah says in the Quran:

> *"O you who believe! Observing As-Saum (the fasting) is prescribed for you as it was prescribed for those before you, that you may become Al-Muttaqun (the pious)."* (Quran 2:183)

And if a Muslim attains Taqwa, he will receive a great reward from Allah,

> *"And march forth in the way (which leads to) forgiveness from your Lord, and for Paradise as wide as are the heavens and the earth, prepared for Al-Muttaqun (the pious)."* (Quran 3:133)

2. Fasting is a means of thanking Allah's blessings

Allah in the verse of fasting of Ramadan:

> *"The month of Ramadan in which was revealed the Quran ...for having guided you so that you may be grateful to Him."* (Quran 2:185)

3. Fasting is a means to do not transgress Allah's limits

Abdullah b. Mas'ud reported that Allah's Messenger said to us:

"O young men, those among you who can support a wife should marry, for it restrains eyes (from casting evil glances) and preserves one from immorality; but he who cannot afford it should observe fast for it is a means of controlling the sexual desire." Muslim (1400)

4. Fasting is a way to attaining forgiveness from Allah

Allah says in Quran:

"Verily, the Muslims (those who submit to Allah in Islam) men and women, the believers men and women (who believe in Islamic Monotheism), the men and the women who are obedient (to Allah), the men and women who are truthful (in their speech and deeds), the men and the women who are patient (in performing all the duties which Allah has ordered and in abstaining from all that Allah has forbidden), the men and the women who are humble (before their Lord Allah), the men and the women who give Sadaqat (i.e. Zakat, and alms, etc.), the men and the women

who observe Saum (fast) (the obligatory fasting during the month of Ramadan, and the optional Nawafil fasting), ... Allah has prepared for them forgiveness and a great reward (i.e. Paradise)." (Quran 33:35)

5. Fasting is a way to get Allah's unlimited reward

Abu Huraira reported Allah's Messenger as saying:

"Allah the Exalted and Majestic said: Every act of the son of Adam is for him, except fasting. It is (exclusively) meant for Me and I (alone) will reward it. Fasting is a shield. When any one of you is fasting on a day, he should neither indulge in obscene language, nor raise the voice; or if anyone reviles him or tries to quarrel with him he should say: I am a person fasting. By Him, in Whose Hand is the life of Muhammad, the breath of the observer of fast is sweeter to Allah on the Day of judgment than the fragrance of musk. The one who fasts has two (occasions) of joy, one when he breaks the fast he is glad with the breaking of (the fast) and one when he meets his Lord he is glad with his fast." Muslim (1151)

This means that the award to fasting is not limited from Allah.

6. Fasting is key to Allah's paradise

The great purpose of every human being is to be one of enters of the Allah's paradise. This paradise that Allah prepared for the pious, he said in his Quran:

"And march forth in the way (which leads to) forgiveness from your Lord, and for Paradise as wide as are the heavens and the earth, prepared for Al-Muttaqun (the pious)." (Quran 3:133)

In Allah's paradise, there is a door called "Ar-Ray-yan" reserved only for those who observe fasting for the sake of Allah, they will enter from it in the day of Judgement.

The Prophet said:

"In Jannah (Paradise) there is a gate which is called Ar-Rayyaan through which only those who observe Saum (fasting) will enter on the Day of Resurrection. None else will enter through it. It will be called out, "Where are those who observe fasting?" So they will stand up and proceed towards it. When the last of them will have en-

tered, the gate will be closed and then no one will enter through that gate." Muslim (1152)

And The Prophet said:

"Paradise has eight gates, and one of them is called Ar-Rayyaan through which none will enter but those who observe fasting." Sahih Al-Bukhari (3257)

7. Fasting is a protection against illnesses and diseases

All studies prove that fasting is an impregnable fortress for many diseases; this is what the Prophet Muhammad referred to fourteen centuries ago:

Abu Huraira reported Allah's Messenger as saying:

"Allah the Exalted and Majestic said: Every act of the son of Adam is for him, except fasting. It is (exclusively) meant for Me and I (alone) will reward it. Fasting is a shield..." Muslim (1151)

In addition to all these reasons and advantages that prompt the Muslim to fast, fasting also achieves the following:

- Seeking nearness to Allah
- A means of intercession on the day of Judgement
- A means of expiating sin
- Acceptance of supplication
- A Following of the practices of the former Allah's messengers...etc.

In addition, Allah has singled out the fast of the month of Ramadan with unique and great benefits, indicates that Allah instituted fasting for great purposes. Among these advantages, which drive to stick to fasting more and more.

1. Month of the descent of the Quran from Allah

Allah says in Quran:

"The month of Ramadan in which was revealed the Quran, a guidance for mankind and clear proofs for the guidance and the criterion (between right and wrong)..." (Quran 2:185)

In the month of Ramadan:

2. The gates of heavens are opened

3. The gates of Hell are closed

4. Every devil is chained up

5. A night which is better than a thousand months (The night of Decree)

It was narrated that Abu Huraira said:

> *"The Messenger of Allah said: 'There has come to you Ramadan, a blessed month, which Allah, the Mighty and Sublime, has enjoined you to fast. In it the gates of heavens are opened and the gates of Hell are closed, and every devil is chained up. In it Allah has a night (The night of Decree) which is better than a thousand months; whoever is deprived of its goodness is indeed deprived."* Sunan an-Nasa'i (2106)

6. The month of forgiveness of sins

Allah's Messenger said:

> *"Whoever observes fasts during the month of Ramadan out of sincere faith, and hoping to attain Allah's rewards, then all his past sins will be forgiven."* Sahih Al-Bukhari (38)

This is in addition to many other advantages of fasting in general and fasting in Ramadan in particular.

Day after day, medical, social and psychological studies prove the validity of all the above mentioned in this book, and emphasizes that fasting in its Islamic form, illustrated by the Quran and the Prophet Muhammad's sayings and deeds, is the greatest and most useful fasting at all (This is main subject of our second book).

CHAPTER VI

How should we fast?

The proper fasting is that fast which must have positive results on the fasting person (man or women) depending on the purpose of fasting. The quran and the prophet Muhammad give us the ultimate way to achieve this fast. The following are all the fundamentals for fasting a one day:

1. The intention

There is agreement among Muslim scholar that the center of intention is the heart. Whatever a person wants to do and for what reason and for the sake of whom will be known by none but all the al-knower. In fasting, intention is determined by the heart seeking to please Allah and obeying his commands.

The Allah's messenger said:

"Actions are to be judged only by intentions and a man will have only what he intended…" Sunan Abi Dawud (2201)

2. Refraining from dawn to sunset

Allah said in his Quran:

"…and eat and drink until the white thread (light) of dawn appears to you distinct from the black thread (darkness of night), then complete your Saum (fast) till the nightfall…" (Quran 2:187)

3. Avoid all that invalidates fasting

Some of these invalidates is having

- ✓ Sexual intercourse
- ✓ Intentional ejaculation of sperm by any means such as masturbation

- ✓ Eating and drinking either it is useful or harmful such as smoking
- ✓ Using injection for nutrition
- ✓ Injection of blood
- ✓ Menstruation or post-natal bleeding
- ✓ Releasing blood by cupping
- ✓ Vomiting deliberately...etc.

Allah says:

"It is made lawful for you to have sexual relations with your wives on the night of As-Saum (the fasts). They are Libas [i.e. body cover, or screen, or Sakan, (i.e. you enjoy the pleasure of living with her), for you and you are the same for them. Allah knows that you used to deceive yourselves, so He turned to you (accepted your repentance) and forgave you. So now have sexual relations with them and seek that which Allah has ordained for you (offspring), and eat and drink until the white thread (light) of dawn appears to you distinct from the black thread (darkness of night), then complete your Saum (fast) till the nightfall..." (Quran 2:187)

Fasting person should observe also all type of obligatory tasks; he should keep away from prohibited matters. He should perform five times prayers in due time in congregation. He should avoid all type of prohibited or disliked things, such as back biting, telling of lie, cheating or taking interest. The prophet Muhammad said:

"Whoever does not give up false statements (i.e. telling lies), and evil deeds, and speaking bad words to others, Allah is not in need of his (fasting) leaving his food and drink." Sahih al-Bukhari (6057)

With all these fundaments of fasting, how should we fast?

The Messenger of Allah (Muhammad) gives us the ultimate response.

1. The intention of fasting

It is essential to make the intention to fast at night, before Fajr. It is not sufficient to start fasting it that day without the intention.

The Allah's messenger said:

"Actions are to be judged only by intentions and a man will have only what he intended..." Sunan

Abi Dawud (2201)

2. Having pre-down meal (suhoor)

Suhoor is the eating and drinking at the end of night with the intention of fasting, the time of suhoor is starts from midnight and ends a few minutes before Fajr (the Dawn), for example, for me if the pre-dawn (fajr) call to prayer (adhan) is at 04 AM, I stop eating and drinking at 3:45 AM.

The Allah's messenger ordered to take suhoor, as he said:

"Suhoor is a blessed meal, so do not omit it, even if one of you only takes a sip of water, for Allaah and His angels send blessings on those who eat suhoor." Saheeh al-Jaami' (3683)

The best time for suhoor is indicated in the narration of Zayd ibn Thaabit that he said:

"We ate suhoor with the Prophet (peace and blessings of Allah be upon him) then he went to pray." I [the narrator] asked, "How long was there between the adhaan (Prayer Call) and suhoor?" He said, "As long as it takes to recite fifty verses."

Al-Bukhaari (1921) and Muslim (1097)

Suhoor meal should be healthy and complete and consist of beneficial nutrients to the body. Foods that contain fat, hot or salty foods should be avoided because they adversely affect the body during the day of fasting.

It's a good idea to include dates, protein sources, and antioxidants hydrating vegetables and drinks in your Suhoor meal.

The fasting person may clean his teeth by using stick (miswak) or brush.

3. Breaking the fast hastily with fresh/ dried dates or water

The Allah's Messenger recommended to hastening in breaking, he said:

"The people will continue to do well so long as they hasten to break the fast." Al-Bukhaari (1957) and Muslim (1098)

Also, Allah loves the person who breaks his fast in its early time, the prophet Muhammad said:

> *"Allah Almighty said: The most beloved among my servants are those who are quickest to break their fast."* Sunan al-Tirmidhi (700)

The ultimate for the fasting person to break his fast is with a few fresh dates, if that is not available, with dry dates, if that is not available, with water.

> *"The Messenger of Allah (blessings and peace of Allah be upon him) used to break his fast with fresh dates before praying. If no fresh dates were available, he would break his fast with dried dates, and if none were available, he would break his fast with a few sips of water."* Abu Dawood (2356) and At-Tirmidhi (696)

There is a very subtle reason why the Prophet would break his fast with fresh dates, or dried dates, or water, because when one fasts, the stomach becomes devoid of nourishment, so the liver will not find anything in the stomach that it can absorb and send to other parts of the body. Sweetness is the quickest to reach the liver and is what it prefers, especially if it is fresh, so if a person eats fresh dates, they will be absorbed quickly by the liver, which will benefit it and other parts of the body. If fresh dates are not available, then dried dates are the next best thing, because they are sweet and nourishing. If there are no dates available, then a few sips of water will extinguish the flame of the stomach and the heat of fasting, thus preparing the stomach to accept food with ease.

Many recently studies have given a very strong proof of this method of breaking the fast, and considered it the most beneficial method of the body at all.

Also, In order to preserve our bodies and make the most of our fasting, the Prophet Muhammad guided us to the best way to eat and drink (Eating and drinking manners), which are respectively:

1. Washing hands and mouth before eating

Messenger of Allah said:

"Whoever would like Allah to increase the goodness of his house, should perform ablution (wash hands) when his breakfast is brought to him and when it is taken away." Ibn Majah (3260)

2. Mentioning Allah's Name before eating any

food

Messenger of Allah said:

"When any of you wants to eat, he should mention the Name of Allah in the beginning, (i.e., say Bismillah). If he forgets to do it in the beginning, he should say (I begin with the Name of Allah at the beginning and at the end)." At-Tirmidhi and Abu Dawud

3. Praising Allah for His Graces when eating

If you eat and become full and if you drink and are sated, should praising Allah to that. The Prophet said:

"Whoever eats food and said: Praise is to Allah Who has fed me this and provided it for me without any strength or power on my part, his previous sins will be forgiven." Sunan Ibn Majah (3285)

4. Not being excessive in food and drink during fast

Messenger of Allah said:

"The human does not fill any container that is worse than his stomach. It is sufficient for the son of Adam to eat what will support his back. If this is not possible, then a third for food, a third for drink, and third for his breath." Jami` at-Tirmidhi (2380)

5. Should not eat whilst reclining

As Allah's Messenger said:

"I do not eat while reclining." Sunan Abi Dawud (3769)

❊ ❊ ❊

At the end of this book, I recommend that you expand your knowledge about fasting with the Islamic method, that it is the best.

The view can be simple, but I believe that if you follow the content step by step you will have great results.